Carnivore Keto Recipes

(Poultry Edition)

Prepare the best keto poultry

Sommario

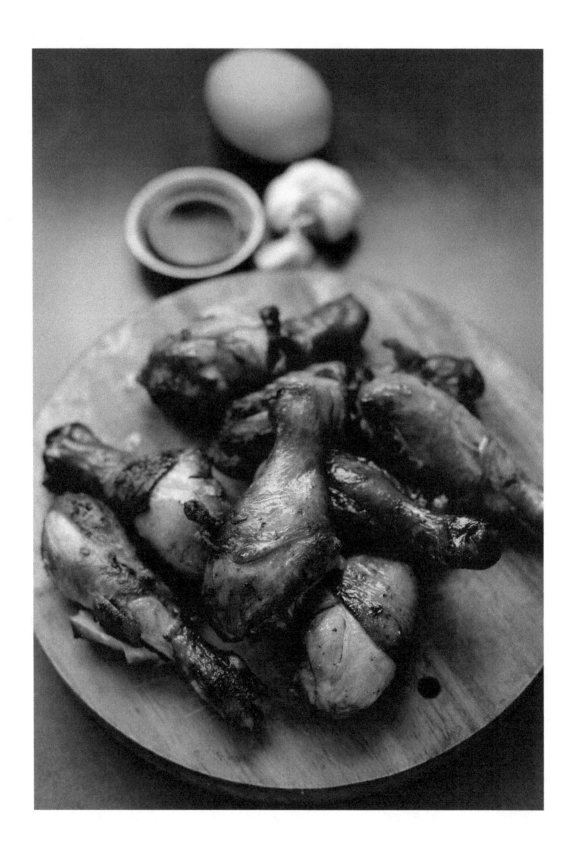

INTRODUCTION

The Keto nutritional regime has always been one of the best and most appreciated!

In this fantastic cookbook we have dedicated ourselves to the most proteinous part of all foods, just poultry.

Chicken has a very high protein intake, with a low amount of fat, so it's perfect for keeping in line but never losing the pleasure of eating delicious dishes.

So let's prepare our poultry together, grab your apron and let's get started right away.

POULTRY RECIPES

262.   <u>CHICKEN-PORK ADOBO</u>

Ingredients

5. 1-kilo pork, cut in 1½" squares

6. 1 head garlic

7. 3 laurel leaves

8. ½ kilo of chicken, cut in serving pieces

9. 8 Tbsp soy sauce

10. 8 Tbsp vinegar

11. 1 Tbsp ground black pepper

12. 1 ½ cup rice water

Instructions

8. In a saucepan, put all the ingredients together.

9. Boil until the chicken and pork are tender.

10. Simmer until the desired consistency of the sauce is reached. Season with soy sauce.

Prep time: 5 min; **Servings:** 4

Macros: 139 Cal 4g Carbs 9g Fat 10g Protein

CHICKEN ADOBO IN COCONUT MILK

Ingredients

- 1 Tbsp oil

- 1 kilo of chicken

- 4 crushed garlic cloves, minced

- 1 potatoes, diced

- 2 cups of rice water

- ½ cup vinegar

- 1 cup thick coconut milk

- Fish sauce (patis)

- 2 bay leaves

- 1 small onion

- Salt to taste

Instructions

1. Saute the garlic and onion in an oiled pan.

2. Add the chicken with a small amount oFish sauce to taste.

3. Add potato, rice water, vinegar, crushed garlic, bay leaves.

4. Cook until chicken is tender.

5. Add coconut milk.

6. Cook over low heat until the desired sauce consistency is reached.

7. Season with salt.

Prep time: 10 min; **Servings:** 2

Macros: 720 Cal 23 g Carbs 53 g Fat 51 g Protein

AFRITADA CHICKEN

Ingredients

- ¼ cup oil

- 1 small potatoes, cubed

- 1 small carrot, cubed

- 2 lb. chicken, cut into bite-sized pieces

- 3 Bay leaves

- 1 small onion, thinly sliced

- 6 garlic cloves, minced

- 2 Tbsp fish sauce

- ¼ tsp ground black pepper

- 1 cup water

- 1 cup tomato sauce

- 1 red bell pepper

- ½ cup green peas, drained

Instructions

1. Heat oil and pan-fry potatoes and carrots lightly browning over medium heat. Set aside.

2. Sear the chicken in the same pan and brown lightly on each side. Set aside.

3. Remove excess oil from the pan, leaving approximately 2 Tbsp.

4. Saute the garlic and onion until fragrant and translucent.

5. Return the seared chicken to the dish, then add the fish sauce and ground black pepper, stirring occasionally for 3 min

6. Pour the water and tomato sauce into the bay leaves, then stir to mix the ingredients.

7. Cover, reduce heat to low and occasionally stir until the chicken is tender and the sauce thickens (about 20-25 min).

8. Add potatoes, carrots, bell peppers and green peas to the dish, cover, and cook for 7 min or until tender.

Prep time: 10 min; **Servings:** 1

Macros: 245 Cal 12g Carbs 9g Fat 28g Protein

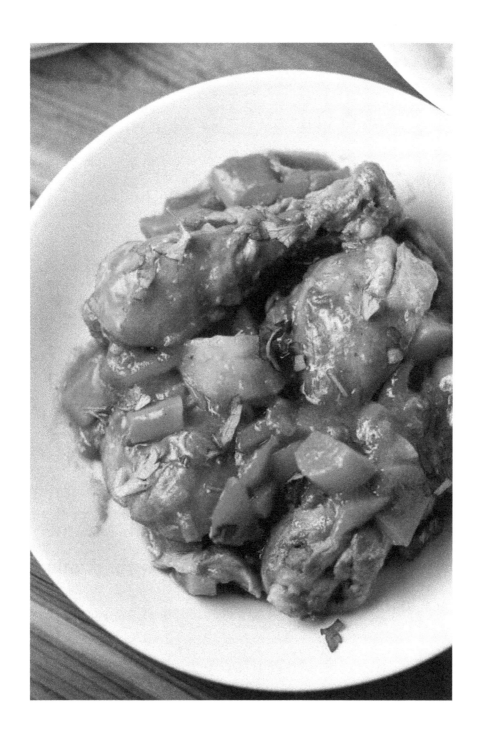

SIMPLE SHEET PAN CHICKEN AND VEGGIES

Ingredients

- 1 (0.7-oz) packet Italian dressing mix

- 1 lb baby carrots

- 1 lb baby Yukon Gold potatoes

- 2 Tbsp olive oil

- 4 to 6 boned chicken thighs with skin

- 8 oz French green beans

- 2 Tbsp butter (optional)

Instructions

1. Preheat oven to 400° ° F. Keep the 1 Tbsp Italian dressing mixture. Combine carrots, onions, oil, and the rest of the dough on a baking sheet covered with aluminum foil and place in a single layer.

2. Sprinkle the chicken with the reserved vinaigrette mixture over the carrot and potato mixture.

3. Bake the chicken in a heated oven until golden and place a thermometer in the thickest part at 35 ° C, 35 to 40 min

4. Add the beans to the potato and carrot mixture. Add the chicken to the vegetable baking sheet. Bake in the oven until the beans are tender and crisp at 400° ° For about 7 min Shake vegetables with butter if desired and serve with chicken.

Prep time:5 min; **Servings:** 4 to 6

Macros: 290 Cal 26g Carbs 14g Fat 18g Protein

CHICKEN INASAL

Ingredients

- 1-kilo chicken; breast and wings preferred

- 4 stalks lemongrass; julienned

- Ground black pepper

- 2 Tbsp 7-up or Sprite

- 1 lemon; juice extracted

- Skewers for grilling

- Salt to taste

- cooking oil

- 4 cloves garlic, crushed

- 1 lime, juice extracted

- 2 Tbsp butter, ¼ cup annatto seeds, Chili pepper flakes (optional)

Instructions

1. Marinate chicken in salt, pepper, garlic, lemongrass, lime and lemon juice, and 7-up or Sprite soda overnight in a pan. Put it aside.

2. In cooking oil, fry annatto seeds. Let the annatto oil cool, crush, and drain in a pan. Put it aside.

3. By adding annatto oil, marinade, and butter, prepare a bashing mixture. Boil the pan for a few min and, if necessary, season with salt and MSG. Sometimes the Philippines have this tantra lang (estimate and approximate) cooking method. Experiment with your best combination, therefore.

4. Squeeze the chicken over the hot charcoal, brushing it once in a while with the mixture. Grill until finished.

Macros: 193 Cal 0g Carbs 8g Fat 26g Protein

Prep time: 10 min; **Servings:** 6

FRIED MARINATED CHICKEN

Ingredients

- Cooking oil

- 1-kilo chicken; cut into desired pieces

- 6 Tbsp fish sauce (patis)

- ¼ Tbsp ground black pepper

- 1 lemon

Instructions

1. Mix fish sauce, pepper and lemon juice and marinate chicken for 3 hours.

2. Deep fry until golden brown in hot cooking oil.

Prep time: 5 min; **Servings:** 4

Macros: 117 Cal 0g Carbs 5g Fat 16g Protein

SIMPLE SLOW COOKER WHOLE CHICKEN

Ingredients

- 1 (4-lb.) whole chicken

- 2 tsp kosher salt

- 1 tsp black pepper

Instructions

1. Remove the neck and giblets of chicken.

2. Sprinkle chicken with salt and pepper.

3. Place in a slow cooker; cover and cook at LOW for 4 hours.

4. Remove and discard the chicken skin and bones and serve.

Prep time: 5 min; **Servings:** 4 to 6

Macros: 159 Cal 1g Carbs 7g Fat 23g Protein

PERFECT PAN-SEARED CHICKEN BREASTS

Ingredients

- 4 (6-oz) skinless, boneless chicken breast halves

- 1 tsp kosher salt

- ½ tsp freshly ground black pepper

- 1 Tbsp canola oil

- 1 tsp butter

Instructions

1. With paper towels, thoroughly dry chicken and season with salt and pepper all over. Put the chicken on a tray in a rimmed baking sheet. Refrigerate for 30 minutes or overnight, uncovered.

2. Heat oil over medium-low heat in a 12-inch straight-sided sauté pan.

3. Cook chicken for 9 min without turning.

4. Apply butter to chicken and underneath.

5. Turn chicken; cook for 6 min or until it reaches an internal temperature of 155°

Prep time:20 min; **Servings:** 4

Macros: 231 Cal 1g Carbs 7g Fat 40g Protein

BUFFALO CHICKEN PIZZA

Ingredients

- Vegetable cooking spray

- ½ cup Buffalo-style hot sauce

- 1 (16-oz) package pre baked Italian pizza crust

- 2 cups chopped deli-roasted whole chicken

- 1 cup (4 oz) shredded Provolone cheese

- ¼ cup crumbled blue cheese

Instructions

1. Coat the grill with the spray and put it on the grill. Preheat grill to 350° F (medium heat).

2. Spread the hot sauce over the crust, and the next 3 ingredients surface.

3. Place the crust on the cooking grate directly. Grill at 350° (medium heat) for 4 min, covered with the grill lid. Rotate 1-

quarter turn pizza and grill, covered with grill top, for 5 to 6 min or until heated thoroughly. Serve right away.

Prep time: 10 min; **Servings:** 5

Macros: 365 Cal 42g Carbs 11g Fat 24g Protein

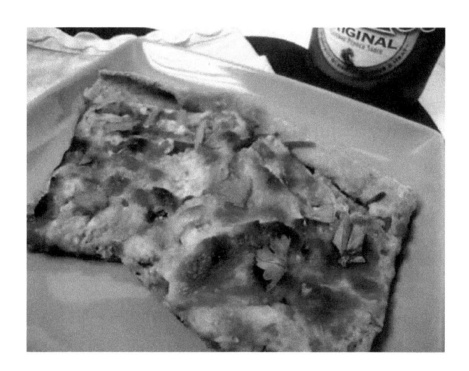

CRISPY OVEN-FRIED DRUMSTICKS

Ingredients

- 3 cups corn flakes cereal, crushed

- ½ tsp salt

- ¼ to ½ tsp ground red pepper

- ¼ tsp freshly ground black pepper

- ⅓ cup grated Parmesan cheese

- 3/4 cup fat-free buttermilk

- 8 chicken drumsticks (about 2 lb.), skinned

- Vegetable cooking spray

Instructions

1. In a large plastic freezer bag, mix the first 5 ingredients; seal and shake well to blend.

2. In a shallow bowl, add buttermilk. Dip 2 buttermilk drumsticks and put them in the bag.

3. Seal and shake well, fully cover drumsticks.

4. Place drumsticks coated with cooking spray on an aluminum foil-lined baking sheet.

5. Repeat with the rest of the drumsticks.

6. Sprinkle the remaining cornflakes mixture on the baking sheet uniformly over drumsticks. Coat lightly with spray for cooking.

7. Also, bake for 25 to 30 minutes at 425° F or until the drumsticks are well browned and finished.

Prep time: 10 min; **Servings:** 6

Macros: 171 Cal 15g Carbs 7g Fat 5g Protein

MESQUITE-SMOKED BEER CAN CHICKEN

Ingredients

- 2 cups mesquite wood chip

- 2 tsp chili powder

- 1 (4-lb) whole chicken

- 1 Tbsp olive oil

- 2 tsp brown sugar

- 1 tsp ground cumin

- 3/4 tsp kosher salt

- ½ tsp black pepper

- 1 (12-oz) can beer

Instructions

1. Soak wood chips in water for 30 minutes; drain well.

2. Use both burners to preheat grill to medium-high heat. Turn off the heater after preheating (leave the right heater on).

3. Pierce the bottom of an aluminum foil pan with a knife's tip. Place the container on the heating element on the grill side; add the wood chips to the pan.

4. Remove from the chicken giblets and back, and discard. Beginning at the cavity of the chest, the skin is loosened from the breasts and drumsticks by inserting fingertips, pressing gently between skin and meat.

5. Combine oil in a bowl with the next 5 ingredients. Rub spice mixture on drumsticks and breasts under loosened skin; let stand for 20 min

6. Holding the chicken body cavity upright, pour the beer into the hole. Place the chicken upright on the grill rack over the left burner and spread the legs to form a tripod. Cover and grill for 1 ½ hours or until it reaches an internal temperature of 165° F.

Prep time:40 min; **Servings:** 4

Macros: 375 Cal 3g Carbs 17g Fat 51g Protein

SLOW COOKER CHICKEN CACCIATORE

Ingredients

- 2 cloves garlic (minced)

- ½ large onion (diced)

- 1 large red bell pepper (diced)

- 1 (14.5 oz) can diced tomatoes (drained)

- 1 Tbsp fresh rosemary (chopped)

- 1 Tbsp fresh thyme (chopped)

- 4 medium chicken breasts

- 1 tsp sea salt

- ¼ tsp black pepper

- 1 medium bay leaf

Instructions

1. Season the chicken fillets with salt and pepper. Put the chicken in the slow cooker.

2. Mix the garlic, onion, pepper, diced tomatoes, rosemary and thyme in a medium bowl. Pour the sauce evenly over the chicken.

3. Place a sheet in the middle of the oven.

4. Cover and cook 3 to 4 hours on high or 6 to 8 hours at low temperature.

5. Serve as quickly as possible. If you want a thicker sauce, remove the chicken and simmer the sauce for another hour in the slow cooker.

Servings: 4; **Prep time:** 10 min

Macros: Cal203 Fat3g Protein 29g Total Carbs 10g Net Carbs 8g Fiber2g Sugar5g

CRISPY AIR FRYER CHICKEN WINGS

Ingredients

- 2 lb chicken wings

- 1 Tbsp baking powder

- 3/4 tsp Sea salt

- ¼ tsp Black pepper

Instructions

1. Combine baking powder, sea salt, and black pepper in a large bowl.

2. Grease 2 frying ovens.

3. Place the wings on the greased trays or place enough arms in the basket to form a single layer. (If you are using a pan, you may need to cook in 2 portions.)

4. Place the bucket or grill in the fryer and bake at 250 For 15 min

5. Turn the wings and turn the drawers upwards and vice versa. Increase the temperature to 430 F (or your deep fryer is the highest).

6. Bake in the oven until the chicken wings are ready and crisp for about 15 to 20 min

Servings: 4; **Prep time:**10 min

Macros: Cal275 Fat19g Protein 22g Total Carbs 1g Net Carbs 1g

KETO CHICKEN ENCHILADAS

Ingredients

- 2 cups gluten-free enchilada sauce

- Chicken

- 1 Tbsp Avocado oil

- 4 cloves Garlic (minced)

- 3 cups Shredded chicken (cooked)

- ¼ cup Chicken broth

- ¼ cup fresh cilantro (chopped)

Assembly

- 12 Coconut tortillas

- 3/4 cup Colby jack cheese (shredded)

- ¼ cup Green onions (chopped)

Instructions

1. Heat oil over medium to high heat in a large pan. Add the chopped garlic and cook until fragrant for about a minute.

2. Add rice, 1 cup enchilada sauce (half the total), chicken, and coriander. Simmer for 5 min

3. In the meantime, heat the oven to 375 F. Grease a 9x13 baking dish.

4. In the middle of each tortilla, place ¼ cup chicken mixture. Roll up and place seam side down in the baking dish.

5. Pour the remaining cup enchilada sauce over the enchiladas. Sprinkle with shredded cheese.

6. Bake for 10 to 12 min Sprinkle with green onions.

Servings: 6; **Prep time:**20 min

Macros: Cal349 Fat19g Protein 31g Total Carbs 17g Net Carbs 9g Fiber 8g Sugar 3

GREEK CHICKEN BOWLS

Ingredients

- 1 lb chicken breast

- 1 ½ tsp Sea salt

- 3 Tbsp Olive oil

- 1 Tbsp Balsamic vinegar (optional)

- ½ tsp Black pepper (divided)

- 2 ½ cups Zucchini (thinly sliced into, ¼ inch thick)

- ½ lb Grape tomatoes

- ½ large onion

- ¼ cup Feta cheese

- ½ Tbsp dried dill

- ½ Tbsp Dried parsley

- 1 tsp dried oregano

- 1 tsp Garlic powder

Instructions

1. Preheat the oven to 400° F. Grease a large baking sheet.

2. Fill a large bowl with water. Add salt and stir to dissolve. Add the chicken and set aside for 10 to 20 min to brine.

3. Chop zucchini, grape tomatoes, and onions.

4. Stir the dried dill, parsley, oregano, garlic powder, salt and pepper in a small bowl.

5. Stick together but not touching when the chicken is cooked, brin, pat dry, and put in 1 region of the baking sheet.

6. Rub a spoonful of olive oil into both sides of the chicken. Season with half the herb mixture.

7. Toss the chopped vegetables and 2 Tbsp olive oil in a large bowl. Add the remaining herb mixture. Toss well to mix. Set the veggies on the baking sheet in a single layer.

8. Roast in the oven for about 20 min

9. Sprinkle with feta cheese (optional)

Servings: 4; **Prep time:**20min

Macros: Cal287 Fat15g Protein 28g Total Carbs 7g Net Carbs 6g Fiber 1g Sugar 4g Cal287

CREAMY GARLIC CHICKEN THIGHS

Ingredients

7. 1 ⅓ lb boneless skinless chicken thighs

8. ½ tsp Sea salt

9. ¼ tsp of smoked paprika

10. A pinch of of Black pepper

11. 2 Tbsp butter (divided)

12. ½ head Garlic

13. ½ cup chicken bone broth

14. ½ cup white cooking wine

15. ¼ cup Heavy cream

16. 1 medium Bay leaf

Instructions

1. Season the chicken with salt, pepper, and smoked paprika on both sides.

2. Heat 1 Tbsp butter over medium heat in a large skillet or skillet. Add the chicken and brown until golden and cooked 5 to 7 min per side.

3. Remove the chicken from the pan and cover with aluminum foil.

4. Put the remaining Tbsp butter in the pan. Add the sliced garlic. Fry until the garlic is fragrant and begins to brown for 2-3 min, stirring frequently.

5. Remove the bread and wine from the pan. Use a wooden spoon to scrape away any brown parts (called enamel) from below.

6. Place the bay leaf in the pan and immerse yourself. Gently bring the liquid to a boil, then increase the heat and cook for 8 to 12 min

7. Turn off heat and put the cream in the hot pan for a few min

8. Serve the chicken with the sauce.

Servings: 4; **Prep time:**5 min

Macros: Cal297 Fat17g Protein 30g Total Carbs 1g Net Carbs 1g

KETO KETO GLUTEN-FREE CHICKEN AND DUMPLINGS

Ingredients

- 1 Tbsp Olive oil

- ½ large Onion

- 1 large Carrot

- 1 stalk Celery

- 2 tsp Italian seasoning

- 1 ½ lb Chicken breast

- 8 cups Chicken broth

- 2 medium Dried bay leaves

- ½ Fathead bagel dough

Instructions

1. Heat olive oil, and saute potatoes, onions, and celery for about 10 min

2. Add Italian seasoning, chicken, chicken broth, and Bay leaves. Cook 6 min in pressure cooker.

3. While, use the same instructions and quantities as the fathead bagels to make fathead bread, except to break the method in half. (Either enter "3" in the bagel serving box, OR make the whole dough, but use only half of it for keto chicken and dumplings.)

4. If the dough is soft, refrigerate until firm for approximately 20 min

5. Place the fathead dough between 2 parchment paper pieces. Roll out, about ¼ in (.5 cm) thick, to a rectangle. Cut into strips with a width of about 2 in (5 cm)x ½ in (1 cm).

6. Remove the lid when the soup is done, and pressure is released. Remove leaves from the harbor.

7. Cut the chicken and cut into bite-sized pieces.

8. Set the Saute mode to the Instant Pot again. Disable for approximately 3 min before cooking.

Servings: 8; **Prep time:** 20 min

Macros: Cal 273 Fat14g Protein 28g Total Carbs 5g Net Carbs 4g Fiber

ADOBONG MANOK SA

Ingredients

- 1-kilo chicken; cut into desired pieces

- 4 cloves garlic; crushed

- 1 small onion; minced

- 1 potato; quartered (optional)

- 1 bell pepper; sliced (optional)

- 2 cups of rice water

- ½ cup vinegar

- 1 cup thick coconut milk

- Fish sauce (patis)

- 2 bay leaves

- Salt to taste

- Cooking oil

Instructions

1. Fry the chopped garlic and onion in an oil pan.

2. Add the chicken until golden brown with a small amount oFish sauce to taste.

3. Add the rice water, vinegar, crushed garlic, bay leaves.

4. Cook until the chicken is tender.

5. Add coconut milk.

6. Simmer and season with salt.

Servings: 8; **Prep time:**10 min

Macros: Cal 243 Fat 12g Protein 25g Total Carbs 4g Net Carbs 4g Fiber 1g

PERFECT PAN-SEARED CHICKEN BREASTS

Ingredients

- 4 (6-oz) skinless, boneless chicken breast halves

- 1 tsp kosher salt

- ½ tsp freshly ground black pepper

- 1 Tbsp canola oil

- 1 tsp butter

Instructions

1. With paper towels, thoroughly dry chicken; season with salt and pepper all over. In a rimmed baking sheet, put the chicken on a rack. Refrigerate, uncovered, for a total of 30 min or overnight. Remove from the fridge; dry pat again.

2. Heat oil over medium-low in a 12-inch straight sauté pan until oil shimmers. Cook for 9 min or until lightly golden brown, without turning.

1. Add the butter; turn, and cover the chicken, so the butter drips down. Bake 1 minute or until golden brown.

2. Turn the chicken over; Broil for 6 min or until a thermometer in the middle of the chest registers 155 ° F. Remove the pan from the heat; Leave the chicken in the pan for 3 min

Prep time:20 min **Servings:** 4

Macros: Cal 128 Fat 8g Protein 11g Net Carbs 1g

COCONUT CURRY CHICKEN

Ingredients

- 4 halves of boneless chicken fillet

- 3 Tbsp melted butter

- 1 cup dried or sweetened unsweetened grated coconut.

- 2 tsp curry powder

- Salt

Instructions

1. Rinse and dry the chicken. Melt the butter into a 9 x 13-inch baking dish. Combine coconut and curry powder in a shallow bowl. Dip the chicken in the butter to cover, then roll in the coconut. Place the slightly separated chicken pieces in the baking dish. Pat the rest of the coconut mixture on top. Sprinkle with salt.

2. Bake the chicken in the oven at 350° For 20 to 25 min

Prep time:30 min; **Servings:** 4

Macros: Cal 190 Fat 13g Protein 17g Net Carbs 3g

CRISPY OVEN-FRIED DRUMSTICKS

Ingredients

- 3 cups of ground cornflakes

- ⅓ cup grated parmesan

- ½ tsp salt

- ¼ to ½ tsp ground red pepper

- ¼ tsp freshly ground black pepper

- 3/4 cup lean serum

- 8 chicken legs (about 2 lbs), skinless

- Spray for cooking vegetables

Instructions

9. Mix the first 5 ingredients in a large plastic bag; close tightly and shake to combine.

10. Pour the whey into a shallow bowl. Dip 2 drumsticks in buttermilk and put them in the bag. Close and stir well and cover the drumsticks well.

11. Place the drumsticks on a baking sheet covered with aluminum foil.

12. sprinkle the remaining cornflakes mixture evenly on a baking sheet on pestles. Lightly coat with cooking spray.

13. Bake for 25 to 30 minutes at 425° F or until the drumsticks are golden and ready.

Prep time: 15 min; **Servings:** 4

Macros: Cal 227 Fat 7g Protein 31g Net Carbs 9g

MAPLE DIJON CHICKEN SKILLET

Ingredients

- 2 large boneless, skinless chicken breasts sliced horizontally to create 4 thin fillets.

- Olive oil

- 1 lb fingerling potatoes, unpeeled, halved lengthwise.

- ¼ tsp salt.

- 3 Tbsp water.

- Spice Rub.

- 1 tsp EACH salt, dried basil, paprika.

- ½ tsp EACH garlic powder, onion powder.

- ¼ tsp EACH pepper, dried thyme.

- Dijon Maple Sauce.

- 3 garlic cloves minced.

- 3 Tbsp Dijon mustard.

- 1 ½ Tbsp pure maple syrup.

- ⅓ cup heavy cream.

- 3/4 cup reduced-sodium chicken broth.

- 3 cups baby spinach.

- Garnish (optional).

- Feta cheese.

- Fresh parsley.

- Crumbled bacon.

Instructions

1. Add potatoes to a microwave-safe dish and add 3 Tbsp water and ¼ tsp salt. Cover and microwave for 5 min

2. In a medium bowl, whisk all the Spice Rub ingredients together. Add 1 Tbsp olive oil to the remaining spices. Add the chicken and rub until uniformly covered with spices.

3. Heat 1 tsp olive oil over medium heat in a 12-inch saucepan until hot. Add the chicken and cook for 2-3 min until golden brown on the bottom, turn them over, cover and reduce heat to medium and cook 3-4 min or until well cooked.

4. With the remaining juices/oil in the now-empty skillet, heat 1 Tbsp olive oil over medium-high heat. Add garlic and potatoes and saute for 1 minute. Add Dijon, maple syrup, heavy cream, chicken broth, and spices that are reserved. Simmer until the sauce has thickened and cooked vegetables. Stir in the spinach and cook for about 30 seconds until just wilted.

5. Add the chicken and warm it up. Garnish with (optional) feta, bacon, and fresh parsley.

Prep time: 10 min; **Servings:** 4

Macros: Cal 277 Fat 3g Protein 34g Net Carbs 38g

HEIRLOOM TOMATO AND CHICKEN TOSS

Ingredients

- 4 Tbsp white wine vinegar

- 3 Tbsp extra-virgin olive oil

- 2 ½ tsp granulated sugar

- 1 ½ tsp kosher salt

- ½ tsp black pepper

- 3 cups shredded cooked chicken

- 2 lbs heirloom tomatoes, cut into ½- to 1-inch wedges

- ½ cup thinly sliced red onion

- 2 Tbsp chopped fresh basil

- 2 Tbsp finely chopped fresh chives

- 2 Tbsp chopped fresh flat-leaf parsley leaves

- 1 Tbsp chopped fresh thyme

Instructions

1. Whisk together vinegar, olive oil, sugar, salt, and pepper in a small bowl.

2. Gently toss together chicken, tomatoes, onions, basil, chives, parsley, and thyme in a large bowl.

3. Add vinegar mixture and gently stir until thoroughly combined.

Prep time: 20 min; **Servings:** 6

Macros: Cal 35 Fat 1g Protein 1g Net Carbs 7g

CHICKEN-AND-BISCUIT COBBLER

Ingredients

- 3 Tbsp butter

- 1 cup sliced carrots

- 1 medium onion, chopped

- 2 (8-oz) packages fresh mushrooms, quartered

- 2 garlic cloves, minced

- ½ cup dry white wine

- ⅓ cup all-purpose flour

- 3 cups reduced-sodium chicken broth

- 3/4 cup whipping cream

- 1 Tbsp white wine vinegar

- 3 Tbsp sliced chives

- 3 Tbsp chopped parsley

- 2 tsp chopped the rosemary

- 2 tsp cut thyme leaves

- 8 cups shredded cooked chicken

- Kosher salt

- Freshly ground black pepper

- 2 ½ cups self-rising flour

- ½ tsp sugar

- 1 ¼ cups chilled buttermilk

- ½ cup butter, melted

- ½ cup chopped cooked bacon.

- Garnishes: chopped fresh chives and parsley

Instructions

1. Preheat the oven to 400° F. Melt butter. Add onion and carrots and sauté for 5 min

2. Stir in mushrooms; sauté for 5 min or until tender. Cut the garlic and sauté for 2 min

3. Add wine and cook for 2 min Sprinkle ⅓ cup all-purpose flour and stir continuously for 3 min

4. Add broth slowly, stirring constantly; bring the mixture to a boil, frequently stirring, for 2 min or until thickened.

5. Add the cream and the next 5 ingredients.

6. Cut the chicken and season with salt and pepper to taste. Protect from the sun and cover it.

7. Whisk 2 ½ cups oFlour and ½ tsp. sugar in a small bowl.

8. Add buttermilk and ½ cup melted butter. Mix buttermilk and bacon in a flour mixture until the dough pulls away from the bowl's edges.

Servings: 8; **Prep time:** 10 min

Macros: Cal 260 Net Carbs 49g Fat 7g Protein 2g

CHICKEN AND FONTINA PANINI

Ingredients

- 1 (8-oz) loaf ciabatta bread, cut in half horizontally

- 3 Tbsp pesto sauce

- 2 plum tomatoes, sliced

- 1 cup shredded rotisserie chicken

- 2 slices fontina cheese

Instructions

5. Preheat panini press.

6. The spread bottom half of bread with pesto. Top with tomato slices, chicken, and cheese. Top with food.

7. Place sandwich in the panini press; cook 3 to 4 min or until cheese melts and bread is toasted. Cut into quarters, and serve hot.

Prep time: 7 min; **Servings:** Serves 2

Macros: Cal 360 Net Carbs 45g Fat 9g Protein 24g

CHICKEN STIR-FRY

Ingredients

6. 1 (14-oz) can low-sodium chicken broth

7. ¼ cup lite soy sauce

8. 1 to 2 Tbsp. chili-garlic sauce

9. 2 Tbsp cornstarch

10. 1 Tbsp brown sugar

11. 1 tsp ground ginger

12. 2 Tbsp dark sesame oil

13. 3 cups shredded rotisserie chicken

14. 1 (16-oz) package frozen stir-fry vegetables

15. Steamed rice

Instructions

1. Mix the chicken broth, soy sauce, yellow chili sauce, cornflour, brown sugar, and ground ginger.

2. Bake 1 to 2 min with chicken and vegetables.

3. Add the broth and cook until the sauce is tender. Serve with steamed rice.

Prep time: 10 min; **Servings:** 4 to 6

Macros: Cal 225 Net Carbs 14g Fat 6g Protein 27g

CHICKEN BREASTS WITH TOMATOES AND OLIVES

Ingredients

- 4 (6-oz) skinless, boneless chicken breast halves.

- 1 cup multicolored cherry or grape tomatoes, halved.

- 3 Tbsp oil and vinegar dressing, divided.

- 20 olives, halved.

- ½ cup (2 oz) crumbled feta cheese.

Instructions

1. Prepare the grill over medium heat. Place the chicken on the rack covered with an oil spray and fry on each side for 6 min or until the chicken is ready. Keep warm

2. Mix the tomatoes, 1 ½ Tbsp sauce, and the olives over medium heat in a medium-sized pan and cook for 2 min or until the vegetables are slightly soft and the mixture is cooked through, stirring occasionally.

3. Brush the chicken with 1 ½ Tbsp the remaining dressing. Cut half of each chicken fillet into 3/4 inch slices. Cover with ¼ cup tomato mixture for each quarter of chicken fillet.

4. If desired, sprinkle with cheese and torn basil leaves.

Prep time: 15 min **Servings:** 4

Macros: Cal 348 Fat 17g Protein 42g Net Carbs 4g

CHICKEN PUTTANESCA WITH ANGEL HAIR PASTA

Ingredients

- 8 oz uncooked angel hair pasta

- 2 tsp olive oil

- 4 (6-oz) skinless, boneless chicken breast halves

- ½ tsp salt

- 2 cups of tomato-basil pasta sauce.

- ¼ cup pitted and coarsely chopped kalamata olives.

- 1 Tbsp capers.

- ¼ tsp crushed red pepper.

- ¼ cup (1 oz) shredded Parmesan cheese.

- Chopped fresh basil or basil sprigs (optional).

Instructions

1. Cook pasta according to the directions of the package, avoiding salt and fat. Drain and stay warm.

2. Heat oil in a large nonstick skillet. Cut the chicken into bits of 1 inch. Place chicken in a saucepan; sprinkle with salt evenly. Cook chicken, occasionally stirring, for 5 min or until lightly browned. Take to boil pasta sauce, olives, capers, and pepper. Cook, frequently stirring, for 5 min or until chicken is finished. Place 1 cup pasta on each of 4 plates; top with a mixture of 1 ½ cups of chicken. Sprinkle 1 Tbsp cheese on each serving. If needed, garnish with sprigs of chopped basil or basil.

Prep time: 10 min

Macros: Cal 530 Fat 12g Protein 57g Net Carbs 55g

BISTRO CHICKEN

Ingredients

6. 2 Tbsp olive oil, divided

7. 4 (6-oz) chicken breast halves, skinned

8. 4 chicken thighs (about 1 lb), skinned

9. 4 chicken drumsticks (about1 lb), skinned

10. 2 cups chopped onion

11. 4 garlic cloves, minced

12. 1 cup chopped celery

13. ½ cup chopped fresh basil

14. ½ cup chopped fresh flat-leaf parsley

15. ½ cup red wine vinegar

16. ¼ cup sliced green olives

17. ¼ cup capers

18. 1 Tbsp sugar

19. Dash of ground red pepper

20. 2 bay leaves

21. 1 (28-oz) can of Italian-style tomatoes, undrained and chopped.

22. 8 cups hot cooked macaroni.

23. Parsley sprigs (optional).

Instructions

1. Heat 1 ½ tsp oil over medium-high heat in a large nonstick skillet. Add the breast half of the chicken to the pan; sauté on each side for 2 min or until lightly brown. Remove from the breadboard. Add 1 ½ tsp oil and remaining pieces of chicken; sauté on each side for 2 min or until lightly browned. Remove the chicken from the casserole.

2. Heat 1 tsp oil in a saucepan. Add garlic and onion; Jump for 5 min Remove the celery; Run for 5 min Apply the basil and the following 8 ingredients (tomato basil). Take the chicken in the pan; bring to a boil. Cover, reduce heat, and cook 20 min

Uncover and simmer for 25 min or until the chicken is tender. Discard bay leaves. Serve with pasta. Garnish with sprigs of parsley, if desired.

Servings: 8; **Prep time:** 15 min

Macros: Cal 20 Fat 0g Protein 1g Net Carbs 4g

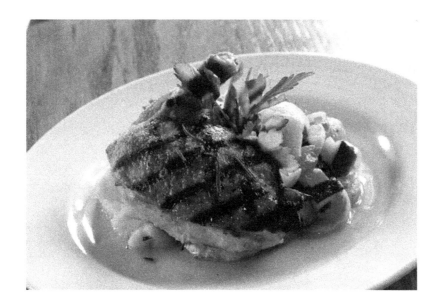

CHICKEN TETRAZZINI

Ingredients

- 1 tsp unsalted butter

- Cooking spray

- 1 cup finely chopped onion

- 2/3 cup finely chopped celery

- 3/4 tsp freshly ground black pepper

- ¼ tsp salt

- 3 packages (8 g) of pre-cut mushrooms

- ½ cup dry sherry

- 3 g of all-purpose flour (about 2/3 cups)

- 3 cans (14.5 oz) fat-free, less-sodium chicken.

- 2 ¼ cups organic Parmesan cheese, grated

- ½ cup (4 oz) cream cheese

- 7 cups hot cooked noodles (about 1 lb of uncooked pasta).

- 4 cups minced grilled chicken fillet (about 1 ½ lbs).

- 1 slice of white bread (1 oz).

Instructions

1. Preheat the oven to 350° F.

2. Melt the butter over medium heat in a big casserole. Add onion, celery, black pepper, salt and mushrooms, cook for 4 min or until tender. Cook for 1 minute. Add the sherry.

3. Weigh or for the flour into dry measuring cups; spirit level with a knife. Gradually add the flour to the pan; Cook for 3 min with continuous stirring (the mixture will be thick) with a whisk. Add the broth slowly, stirring constantly. Bring to a boil. Lower the temperature; simmer 5 minutes, stirring regularly. Remove from fire.

4. Add 1 ¾ cup Parmesan and cream cheese, stir with a whisk until the cream cheese melts. Add pasta and chicken; Stir until everything is mixed. Divide the pasta mixture with an oil spray into 2 8-inch square glass or ceramic baking sheets.

5. Place the bread in a food processor; press 10 times or to form thick crumbs. Combine breadcrumbs and ½ cup Parmesan; sprinkle evenly over the pasta.

6. Bake in the oven at 350° For 30 min or until they are light brown and sparkling.

7. Freezing a frying pan without frying: Prepare step by step. Let cool completely in the refrigerator. Cover and press to remove as much air as possible with plastic wrap. Use a strong sheet to wrap. Store in the freezer for up to 2 months.

Servings: Serves 12 (serving size: about 1 ⅓ cups; 6 Servings: per casserole) **Prep time:** 15 min

Macros: Cal 500 Net Carbs 40g Fat 27g Protein26g

CHICKEN SHAWARMA

Ingredients

Chicken:

- 2 Tbsp fresh lemon juice

- 1 tsp curry powder

- 2 tsp extra virgin olive oil

- 3/4 tsp salt

- ½ tsp ground cumin

- 3 garlic cloves, minced

- 1 lb skinless, boneless chicken breast, cut into 16 (3-inch) strips

Sauce:

- ½ cup plain Greek yogurt

- 2 Tbsp tahini

- 2 tsp fresh lemon juice

- ¼ tsp salt

- 1 garlic clove, minced

- Cooking spray

- 4 (6-inch) pitas

- 1 cup chopped romaine lettuce

- 8 (¼-inch) tomato slices

Instructions

5. Preheat grill to medium-high heat.

6. To prepare chicken, combine first 6 ingredients in a medium bowl. Add chicken to pan; toss well to coat. Let stand at room temperature 20 min

7. To prepare sauce, combine yogurt and next 4 ingredients, stirring with a whisk.

8. Thread 2 chicken strips onto each of 8 (12-inch) skewers. Place kebabs on a grill rack coated with cooking spray; grill 4 min on each side or until done.

9. Place pitas on grill rack; grill 1 minute on each side or until lightly toasted. Place 1 pita on each of 4 plates; top each serving with ¼ cup lettuce and 2 tomato slices. Top each meal with 4 chicken pieces; drizzle each meal with 2 Tbsp sauce.

Prep time:45 min; **Servings:** 4

Macros: Cal 430 Net Carbs 45g Fat 9g Protein 39g

CHICKEN, MUSHROOM AND GRUYERE QUESADILLAS

Ingredients

- 1 tsp olive oil

- 1 cup mushrooms

- ½ cup thinly sliced onion

- A pinch of salt

- A pinch of oFreshly ground black pepper.

- 1 tsp minced garlic

- 1 Tbsp sherry or red wine vinegar

- 2 (10-inch) fat-free flour tortillas

- 1 cup shredded chicken breast (about 8 oz)

- 1 cup arugula

- ½ cup (2 oz) shredded Gruyère cheese

Instructions

1. Heat a large skillet over medium-high heat. In a bowl, add olive oil; swirl to coat.

2. Add mushrooms, onion cut, salt, and pepper; sauté for 5 min Cut the garlic and sauté for 30 seconds. Apply vinegar; cook for 30 seconds.

3. Arrange half of each tortilla's mushroom mixture over half. Using ½ cup chicken, ½ cup arugula, and ¼ cup cheese to top each tortilla; fold half of the tortillas.

4. Clean the pan with a paper towel. Over medium heat, coat pan with cooking spray.

5. Cook tortillas on each side for 2 min or until crisp.

Prep time: 20 min **Servings:** 2

Macros: Cal 210 Net Carbs 28g Fat 6g Protein 11g

CHEESE CHICKEN PENNE FLORENTINE

Ingredients

- 1 tsp olive oil

- Cooking spray

- 3 cups thinly sliced mushrooms

- 1 cup chopped onion

- 1 cup chopped red bell pepper

- 3 cups chopped fresh spinach

- 1 Tbsp chopped fresh oregano

- ¼ tsp freshly ground black pepper

- 1 (16-oz) carton cottage cheese

- 4 cups hot cooked penne

- 2 cups shredded the roasted skinless, boneless chicken breast

- 1 cup (4 oz) shredded reduced-fat sharp cheddar cheese.

- ½ cup (2 oz) grated fresh Parmesan cheese

- ½ cup 2% reduced-fat milk

- 1 (10 3/4-oz) can condense reduced-fat, reduced-sodium cream of chicken soup, undiluted

Instructions

1. Preheat oven to 425°.

2. 2. Heat olive oil over medium-high heat in a large nonstick skillet coated with cooking spray. Add mushrooms, onion, and bell pepper; sauté 4 min or until tender. Add spinach, oregano, and black pepper; sauté 3 minutes or just until spinach wilts.

3. Place cottage cheese in a food processor; process until very smooth. Combine spinach mixture, cottage cheese, pasta, chicken, 3/4 cup cheddar cheese, ¼ cup Parmesan cheese, milk, and soup in a large bowl. Spoon mixture into a 2-quart baking dish coated with cooking spray. Sprinkle with remaining ¼ cup cheddar cheese and remaining ¼ cup Parmesan cheese. Bake at 425° for 25 min or until lightly browned and bubbly.

Servings: 8 Servings:; **Prep time:** 20 min

Macros: Cal 345 Net Carbs 33g Fat 10g Protein 32g

CHICKEN STRIPS WITH BLUE CHEESE DRESSING

Ingredients

Chicken:

- ½ cup low-fat whey

- ½ tsp hot sauce

- ½ cup all-purpose flour

- ½ tsp bell pepper

- ½ tsp ground red pepper

- ½ tsp freshly ground black pepper

- ¼ tsp salt

- 1 lb chicken fillet

- 1 Tbsp rapeseed oil

Dressing:

- ½ cup fat-free mayonnaise

- ¼ cup (1 oz) grated cheese

- 1 Tbsp red wine vinegar

- 1 tsp chopped garlic in bottles

- ¼ tsp salt

- ¼ tsp freshly ground black pepper

Instructions

1. To prepare the chicken, mix the whey and the hot sauce on a deep plate.

2. Combine flour and the following 4 ingredients in a shallow bowl. Dip the chicken in the whey mixture and dredge it in flour mixture.

3. Heat the oil in a large skillet over medium heat. Add chicken; Bake 4 min on each side or until cooked through. Remove from the pan. Keep warm.

4. Prepare the dressing while the chicken cooks. Combine the fat-free mayonnaise and the following 5 ingredients in a small bowl.

Prep time:15 min **Servings:** 4

Macros: Cal 500 Net Carbs 0g Fat 3g Protein 8g

POTATO, CHICKEN AND FRESH PEA SALAD

Ingredients

- 1 lb fingerling potatoes, cut crosswise into 1-inch pieces

- 2 cups fresh sugar snap peas

- 2 cups chopped skinless, boneless rotisserie chicken breast

- ½ cup red bell pepper finely chopped

- ½ cup red onion chopped

- 2 Tbsp extra-virgin olive oil

- 2 Tbsp white wine vinegar

- 1 Tbsp fresh lemon juice

- 1 Tbsp Dijon mustard

- 1 tsp minced fresh tarragon

- 1 tsp salt

- ½ tsp freshly ground black pepper

- 1 garlic clove, minced

Instructions

1. Place potatoes in a large saucepan; cover with cold water. Bring to a boil. Reduce heat, and simmer 10 min or until almost tender. Add peas; cook 2 min or until peas are crisp-tender. Drain; place vegetables in a large bowl. Add chicken, bell pepper, and onion.

2. Combine oil and remaining ingredients, stirring with a whisk. Drizzle over salad; toss gently to combine.

Servings: 4 (serving size: about 1 ½ cups); **Prep time:** 30 min

Macros: Cal 316 Net Carbs 29g Fat 9g Protein 28g

CHICKEN SKEWERS WITH SOY-MIRIN MARINADE

Ingredients

- ⅓ cup mirin (sweet rice wine)

- ⅓ cup low-sodium soy sauce

- 1 tsp dark sesame oil.

- 1 ½ lbs skinless, boneless chicken breast halves, cut lengthwise into 1-inch strips.

- 1 large red bell pepper, cut into 8 pieces

- 1 large green bell pepper, cut into 8 pieces

- Cooking spray

- 2 Tbsp sesame seeds, toasted

- 3 cups hot cooked rice

Instructions

1. Combine first 3 ingredients in a large bowl; add chicken and toss to coat. Let stand 15 min, turning chicken occasionally.

2. Prepare grill.

3. Remove chicken from bowl.

4. Place marinade in a small saucepan; bring to a boil. Cook until reduced to ¼ cup (about 5 min). Thread chicken and bell peppers on 8 (12-inch) wooden skewers. Brush skewers with marinade.

5. Place skewers on the grill rack.

6. Grill 4 min on each side, occasionally brushing with remaining marinade. Remove from grill; sprinkle with sesame seeds. Serve with rice.

Prep time: 10 min **Servings:** 4

Macros: Cal 126 Net Carbs 1g Fat 4g Protein 22g

CHICKEN AND CASHEWS

Ingredients

- 3 Tbsp low sodium soy sauce, divided

- 2 dry sherry Tbsp

- 2 tsp cornstarch, divided

- 1 boneless lb, skinless chicken fillet, cut into small pieces

- ½ cup fat-free, less-sodium chicken broth

- 2 Tbsp oyster sauce

- 1 Tbsp honey

- 2 tsp sesame oil, divided

- 3/4 cup chopped onion

- ½ cup chopped celery

- ½ cup chopped red pepper

- 1 Tbsp grated fresh ginger

- 2 finely chopped garlic cloves

- ½ cup chopped green onions (about 3 green onions)

- ¼ cup dry salted dry roasted cashews

Instructions

1. Combine 1 Tbsp soy sauce, sherry, 2 tsp cornstarch, and chicken in a large bowl; toss well to coat. Combine the remaining 2 Tbsp soy sauce, remaining 2 tsp cornstarch, broth, oyster sauce, and honey in a small bowl.

2. Heat 1 tsp oil over medium-high heat in a large nonstick skillet. Add the mixture of chicken to pan; sauté for 3 min

3. Add onion, celery, and bell pepper to pan; sauté 2 min Add ginger and garlic; sauté 1 minute. Return chicken mixture to pan; sauté 1 minute.

4. Stir in broth mixture. Bring to a boil; cook 1 minute, stirring constantly. Remove from heat. Sprinkle with green onions and cashews.

Prep time: 10 min; **Servings:** 6

Macros: Cal 591 Net Carbs 29g Fat 32g Protein 33g

THAI CHICKEN SAUTÉ

Ingredients

- 1 ½ lbs chicken breast tenders

- 1 Tbsp cornstarch

- 1 Tbsp fish sauce

- 4 tsp canola oil, divided

- 1 cup sliced onion

- 2 tsp bottled minced garlic

- • 1 Tbsp fresh ginger bottled soil

- ½ cup coconut milk

- 2 Tbsp Sriracha (hot chili sauce, such as Huy Fong)

- 1 Tbsp sugar

- 1 Tbsp fresh lime juice

- 2 Tbsp chopped fresh cilantro

- 4 lime wedges

Instructions

1. Mix the chicken with the cornmeal and the fish sauce.

2. Heat 1 Tbsp oil in a large nonstick skillet over medium-high heat. Return the chicken to the pan

3. Bake 1 minute or until cooked through.

Prep time: 20 min; **Servings:** 4

Macros: Cal 430 Net Carbs 40g Fat 8g Protein 20g

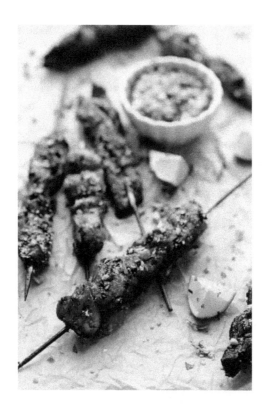

BISCUIT-TOPPED CHICKEN POT PIE

Ingredients

- 1 Tbsp butter

- 2 cups chopped leek

- ¼ cup chopped shallot

- • 3/4 tsp dried thyme chopped fresh or ¼ tsp

- 1 ½ cup diced potatoes chilled with onion (just like potatoes)

- ⅓ cup dry white wine

- 1 tsp Dijon mustard

- 1 can (14 oz) fat-free, less-sodium chicken broth

- 2 cups chopped roasted chicken filet1 ½ cups frozen vegetables

- ¼ tsp salt

- ¼ tsp freshly ground black pepper

- 1 ½ Tbsp cornflour

- 2 Tbsp water

- 2/3 and a half cups

- Cooking spray

- 1 ¼ cups low-fat baking mix (like Bisquick Heart Smart)

- ½ cup skim milk

- 1 abundant lightly beaten protein

Instructions

1. Preheat the oven to 425 °.

2. Melt the butter in a large skillet over medium-high heat. Add the leeks, shallots, and thyme; Skip 2 min Add potatoes; Skip 2 min Add wine; boil 1 minute or until the liquid evaporates. Add mustard and broth; bring to a boil. Cook 4 minutes, stirring occasionally. Add chicken, mixed vegetables, salt, and pepper; Boil for 1 minute Mix cornstarch and 2 Tbsp water in a small bowl, stirring with a whisk. Add the cornflour mixture and 1 and a half and half to the pan. Reduce the heat and simmer for 2 minutes, stirring

constantly. Place the dough in a 13 x 9-inch baking dish covered with an oil spray.

3. Lightly mix the cooking mixture in dry measuring cups; spirit level with a knife. Combine dough mixture, milk, and egg in a medium bowl, stirring with a whisk. Place dough on chicken mixture; Spread evenly to cover. Bake for 20 minutes at 425 ° or until the filling is golden and the filling has bubbles. Let stand for 10 min

Servings: 6(serving size: 1 ½ cups).**Prep time**:20 min

Macros: Cal 350° Net Carbs 27g Fat 23g Protein 10g

BAKED CHICKEN AND BROCCOLI

Ingredients

7. 3 liters of water

8. 1 package (12 g) of broccoli florets

9. 4 boneless, skinless chicken halves

10. 1 (12 oz) can evaporated milk

11. ¼ cup all-purpose flour (about 1 oz)

12. ¼ tsp salt

13. ¼ tsp freshly ground black pepper

14. A pinch of nutmeg

15. 1 cup fat-free mayonnaise

16. ½ cup fat-free sour cream

17. ¼ cup dry sherry

18. 1 tsp Worcestershire sauce

19. 1 (10.75 oz) can mushroom cream, undiluted

20. 1 cup grated fresh Parmesan cheese, divided

21. Cooking spray

Instructions

1. Preheat the oven to 400° F.

2. Boil the water in a large Dutch oven over medium heat. Add the broccoli and cook for 5 min or until it is tender and crisp.

3. Transfer the broccoli to a large bowl with a slotted spoon.

4. Add chicken to boiling water; reduce heat and simmer for 15 min or until cooked. Place the chicken on a cutting board; a little cool. Cut the chicken into small pieces and add to the bowl with the broccoli.

5. Combine evaporated milk, flour, salt, pepper, and nutmeg in a saucepan, stirring in a smooth mixture with a whisk. Bring to a boil over medium heat; Cook for 1 minute with continuous stirring. Remove from fire.

6. Add the mayonnaise, the following 4 ingredients (through the soup) and ½ cup cheese, stirring until well combined. Add the mayonnaise mixture to the broccoli mixture; Stir gently until well blended.

7. Pour the mixture with a spoon into a 13 x 9-inch baking dish covered with oil. Sprinkle with the remaining ½ cup cheese. Bake for 50 min at 400° F or until mixture boils around the edges and the cheese begins to brown. Remove from the oven; let cool on a wire rack for 5 min

Prep time: 25 min; **Servings:** 8

Macros: Cal 284 Net Carbs 16 g Fat 7 g Protein 37 g

FIESTA CHICKEN TACOS WITH MANGO AND JICAMA SALAD

Ingredients

Salad:

- 3/4 cup (3-inch) julienne-cut peeled jicama

- ½ cup sliced peeled ripe mango

- ¼ cup pre sliced red onions

- 1 Tbsp fresh lime juice

- ½ tsp sugar

- 1 ½ tsp chopped fresh cilantro

- ¼ tsp salt

- Dash of black pepper

- Tacos:

- 1 Tbsp olive oil, divided

- 1 lb skinless, boneless chicken breast, cut into thin strips

- ½ tsp chili powder

- ½ tsp ground cumin

- A pinch of ground chipotle chile pepper

- 1 cup pre sliced red bell pepper

- 1 cup pre sliced red onion

- ¼ tsp salt

- 8 (6-inch) corn tortillas

- 1 cup mixed salad greens

Instructions

6. To prepare salad, combine first 8 ingredients.

7. To prepare tacos, heat 2 tsp oil in a large nonstick skillet over medium-high heat. Sprinkle chicken evenly with chili powder, cumin, and chipotle pepper. Remove from pan.

8. Heat remaining 1 tsp oil in a pan. Add bell pepper and 1 cup onion; cook 3 minutes or until crisp-tender. Return chicken mixture to pan; cook 2 min or until chicken is done. Sprinkle with ¼ tsp salt.

9. Heat tortillas according to package directions. Arrange 2 Tbsp mixed greens, about ⅓ cup chicken mixture, and about 2 Tbsp salad in each tortilla; fold over.

10. Heat remaining 1 tsp oil in a pan. Add bell pepper and 1 cup onion; cook 3 minutes or until crisp-tender. Return chicken mixture to pan; cook 2 min or until chicken is done. Sprinkle with ¼ tsp salt.

11. Heat tortillas according to package directions. Arrange 2 Tbsp mixed greens, about ⅓ cup chicken mixture, and about 2 Tbsp salad in each tortilla; fold over.

Prep time: 15 min; **Servings:** 4

Macros: Cal 82 Net Carbs 8g Fat 6g Protein 2g

CHICKEN POT PIE

Ingredients

- 2 butter spoons

- 2 Tbsp olive oil

- 3 cups diced red potato (about 1 lb)

- 2 cups chopped onion

- 2 cups of sliced mushrooms (about 8 g)

- 1 cup diced celery

- 1 cup chopped carrot

- ¼ cup chopped fresh parsley

- 2 chopped fresh thyme tsp

- 6 ½ Tbsp all-purpose flour

- 3 cups of skim milk

- ½ cup fat-free, less-sodium chicken broth

- 2 cups minced cooked chicken fillet (about 12 g)

- 1 cup frozen green peas

- 1 tsp salt

- ½ tsp freshly ground black pepper

- 6 sheets (14 x 9 inches) oFrozen filo pastry, thawed

- Cooking spray

Instructions

1. Preheat the oven to 375 °.

2. Melt the butter in a large Dutch oven over medium heat; add the oil Add the potatoes and the following 6 ingredients (through the thyme) and fry for 5 min Lower the temperature to medium to low; sprinkle the flour over the vegetables.

3. Cook 5 minutes, stirring regularly. Add the milk and broth. Set the heat higher to medium-high; bring to a boil. Reduce heat and simmer 5 min or until thickened. Add the chicken, peas, salt, and pepper.

4. Place the mixture in a 3-quart baking dish. Place 1 cutting edge on a large cutting board or work surface (cover the remaining dough to prevent it from drying out); Lightly spray with spray oil.

5. Repeat the layers with spray oil and the remaining edge. Place the dish on a baking sheet. Bake for 30 minutes at 375 ° or until the top is golden.

Servings: 6 **Prep time:** 25 min

Macros: Cal 310 Net Carbs 36g Fat 13g Protein 20g

ROAST CHICKEN SALAD WITH PEACHES, GOAT CHEESE AND PECANS

Ingredients

- 2 ½ Tbsp balsamic vinegar

- 1 ½ Tbsp extra virgin olive oil

- 1 ½ Tbsp chopped shallots

- 2 ½ tsp fresh lemon juice

- 2 ½ tsp maple syrup

- 3/4 tsp Dijon mustard

- ¼ tsp kosher salt

- ¼ tsp freshly ground black pepper

- 2 cups boneless roasted chicken fillet

- 2 cups peeled sliced peaches

- ½ cup vertically sliced red onion

- ¼ cup chopped walnuts, toasted

- 1 package (5 oz) gourmet vegetable salad

- 2 Tbsp grated goat cheese

Instructions

6. Combine the first 8 ingredients; stir with a whisk.

7. Combine chicken and remaining ingredients except for cheese in a large bowl.

8. Add vinegar mixture; toss gently.

9. Sprinkle with cheese.

Prep time: 30 min; **Servings:** 4

Macros: Cal 160 Net Carbs 18g Fat 6g Protein 11g

CHICKEN-ESCAROLE SOUP

Ingredients

- 1 (14 ½-oz) can Italian-style stewed tomatoes, undrained and chopped

- 1 (14-oz) can chicken broth

- 1 cup chopped cooked chicken breast

- 2 cups coarsely chopped escarole (about 1 small head)

- 2 tsp extra-virgin olive oil

Instructions

1. Combine tomatoes and food in a large saucepan.

2. Cover and bring to a boil over high heat. Reduce heat to low; simmer 5 min

3. Add chicken, escarole, and oil; cook 5 min

Prep time:15 min; **Servings:** 4

Macros: Cal 360 Net Carbs 19g Fat 18g Protein 30g

CHICKEN AND TAMALE CASSEROLE

Ingredients

- 1 cup (4 oz) Mexican cheese premixed with 4 kinds of cheese, divided

- ⅓ cup skim milk

- ¼ cup egg substitute

- 1 tsp ground cumin

- A pinch of ground red pepper

- 1 can (14 3/4 oz) creamy corn

- 1 can (8.5 oz) corn muffin mix (like Martha White)

- 1 (4 g) can chop the green pepper, drained

- Cooking spray

- 1 can (10 oz) red enchilada sauce

- 2 cups grated cooked chicken fillet

- ½ cup fat-free sour cream

Instructions

6. Preheat the oven to 400° F.

7. Combine ¼ cup cheese and the following 7 ingredients (per chili peppers) in a large bowl, stirring until moist. Pour mixture into a 13 x 9-inch baking dish covered with an oil spray.

8. Bake for 15 min Generously pierce with a fork; pour the enchilada sauce over it. Cover with chicken; sprinkle with 3/4 cup cheese. Bake for 15 min at 400° F or until the cheese melts. Remove from the oven; let stand for 5 min Cut into 8 pieces; Cover each serving with 1 Tbsp sour cream.

Prep time: 20 min; **Servings:** 8

Macros: Cal 354 Net Carbs 36 g Fat 14 g Protein 19 g

CHEESY CHICKEN ENCHILADAS

Ingredients

- 2 ½ cups chopped cooked chicken breast

- 2 cups (8 oz) pre-shredded reduced-fat 4-cheese Mexican blend cheese

- 1 2/3 cups plain low-fat yogurt

- ⅓ cup butter, melted

- ¼ cup chopped onion

- 1 tsp minced garlic

- ¼ tsp freshly ground black pepper

- 1 (10 3/4-oz) can condense reduced-fat, reduced-sodium cream of chicken soup (such as Healthy Request), undiluted

- 1 (4.5-oz) can be chopped green chiles, drained

- 8 (8-inch) flour tortillas

- 1 Tbsp canola oil

- Cooking spray

- ½ cup (2 oz) finely shredded reduced-fat sharp cheddar cheese

- ¼ cup chopped green onions

Instructions

7. Preheat oven to 350° F.

8. Combine the first 9 ingredients in a large bowl. Set mixture aside.

9. Heat a large skillet over medium-high heat. Working with 1 tortilla at a time, brush oil on both sides. Remove from pan; arrange ½ cup chicken mixture down the center of the tortilla.

10. Roll jelly-roll style; a place filled tortilla, seam side down, in a 13 x 9-inch baking dish coated with cooking spray. Repeat procedure with remaining 7 tortillas, oil, and chicken mixture. Spread reserved 1 cup chicken mixture evenly over enchiladas.

11. Cover and bake for 20 min Uncover; sprinkle evenly with cheddar cheese and green onions; bake an additional 5 min or until cheese melts.

Prep time:15 min; **Servings:** 8 Servings:

Macros: Cal 267 Net Carbs 32g Fat 8g Protein 16g

CHICKEN VEGETABLE SOUP

Ingredients

- 2 quarts chicken bouillon

- 1 cup sliced carrots

- 1 cup fresh or frozen green peas

- 1 cup chopped celery

- 1 tsp salt

- 2 cups diced cooked chicken

- 1 tsp dried whole rosemary

- 1 tsp dried whole thyme

Instructions

1. Combine first 5 ingredients in a large Dutch oven; bring to a boil.

2. Stir in remaining ingredients. Reduce heat; cover and simmer 15 min or until vegetables are tender.

Prep time: 10 min; **Servings:** 2

Macros: Cal 120 Net Carbs 11g Fat 4g Protein 10g

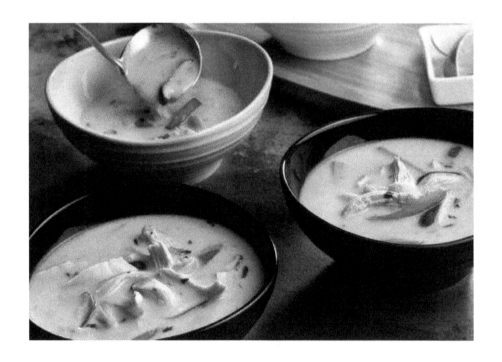

BLACK BEAN AND CHICKEN CHILAQUILES

Ingredients

- Cooking spray

- 1 cup thinly sliced onion

- 5 garlic cloves, minced

- 2 cups shredded cooked chicken breast

- 1 (15-oz) can black beans, rinsed and drained

- 1 cup fat-free, less-sodium chicken broth

- 1 (7 3/4-oz) can fresh chili salsa

- 15 (6-inch) corn tortillas, cut into 1-inch strips

- 1 cup shredded white cheese

Instructions

1. Preheat oven to 450° F.

2. Heat a large nonstick skillet over medium-high heat. Coat pan with cooking spray. Add onion; sauté 5 min or until lightly browned.

3. Add garlic and chicken; sauté 1 minute.

4. Transfer mixture to a medium bowl; stir in beans. Add broth and salsa to pan; bring to a boil. Reduce heat, and simmer for 5 minutes, stirring occasionally. Set aside.

5. Place half of the tortilla strips in the bottom of an 11 x 7-inch baking dish coated with cooking spray.

6. Layer half of the chicken mixture over tortillas; top with remaining tortillas and chicken mixture. Pour broth mixture evenly over chicken mixture. Sprinkle with cheese.

7. Bake for 10 min or until tortillas are lightly browned, and cheese is melted.

Prep time: 10 min; **Servings:** 6

Macros: Cal 293 Net Carbs 40g Fat 5g Protein 23g

GRILLED CHICKEN AND FARFALLE PESTO

Ingredients

- Cut in half 1 3/4 lbs of boneless chicken.

- 1 tsp salt, split, 3/4 tsp black pepper freshly ground, split.

- Spray for cooking.

- Twenty g of untreated farfalle (bow tie paste).

- 1 spoonful of sugar.

- 3 garlic cloves, finely chopped.

- Divided 1 ½ cup 1% skim milk.

- 2 all-purpose flour spoons.

- 1 commercial pesto bottle (3.5 oz) (approximately ⅓ cup).

- Half-and - a-half cup 3/4, ½ cup fresh basil.

- 2 cups oFresh Parmesan grated cheese, 4 cups of half tomatoes (about 2 pints).

Instructions

1. Using medium heat to prepare the grill.

2. Apply ¼ tsp salt and ¼ tsp pepper to the meat. Place the chicken on the grill coated with an oil spray; grill for 10 min or until it is cooked, turning 6 min later. Clear from the grill; allow 5 min to stand. Cut the chicken into pieces of ½ inch; keep warm.

3. Cook pasta, without salt or fat, according to the instructions of the box. Drain over a bowl in a colander and store liquid for ¼ cup cooking. Place the pasta in a large bowl.

4. Heat butter over medium heat in a medium saucepan. Add garlic to the pan; bake for 1 minute, sometimes stirring. In a small bowl, mix ½ cup milk and flour, stir with a whisk. Add the mixture of milk to the oven, stirring constantly with a whisk. Stir in the pesto. Gradually add remaining 1 ½ cups of milk, stirring constantly with a whisk. Bake for 8 min, stirring frequently, or until sauce thickens. Add ¼ cup reserved cooking liquid, 3/4 tsp residual salt, ½ tsp residual pepper and 1 cup of cheese; remove until the cheese melts.

5. Stir well to fill with chicken and pasta sauce. Shake softly with tomatoes and basil. Sprinkle with 1 cup cheese left.

Prep time: 15 min **Servings:** 10

Macros: Cal 508 Net Carbs 51 g Fat 17 g Protein 38 g

CHICKEN SCALOPPINE OVER BROCCOLI RABE

Ingredients

- 1 Tbsp olive oil

- ⅓ cup Italian-seasoned breadcrumbs

- ¼ tsp black pepper

- 4 (6-oz) skinless, boneless chicken breast cutlets

- ½ cup dry white wine

- ½ cup fat-free, less-sodium chicken broth

- 3 Tbsp fresh lemon juice

- 1 tsp butter

- 1 lb broccoli rabe (rapini), cut into 3-inch pieces

- 2 Tbsp chopped fresh parsley

- 2 Tbsp capers, rinsed and drained

- 4 lemon slices (optional)

Instructions

1. Heat the oil in a large nonstick skillet over medium-high heat.

2. Combine breadcrumbs and pepper in a shallow dish; dredge chicken in breadcrumb mixture. Add chicken to pan; cook 3 minutes on each side or until done. Remove from pan; keep warm.

3. Add wine, broth, juice, and butter to the pan, scraping the pan to loosen browned bits.

4. Stir in broccoli rabe; cover and cook 3 min or until broccoli rabe are tender. Stir in parsley and capers. Serve chicken over broccoli rabe mixture. Garnish with lemon slices, if desired.

Prep time:20 min **Servings:** 4

Macros: Cal 318 Net Carbs 14g Fat 7g Protein 44g

CONCLUSION

I'm still licking my lips over these delights and I'm sure you will be delighted by these recipes as well.

Have you had the whole family try them? Are you practicing making them to get better and better at them?

Just keep making them and never stop and you will see excellent results.

I remind you to always consult a nutritionist before embarking on any diet, so that they can advise you on the best way to stay healthy.

Thank you and I embrace you

CPSIA information can be obtained
at www.ICGtesting.com
Printed in the USA
BVHW051756050421
604209BV00009B/655